HERBAL ANTIVIRAL CARE

Fast and Effective Ways to Fight Viruses, Boost Immunity and Keep You Stay Healthy Always

STEPHEN BRIGHT

TABLE OF CONTENT

CHAPTER ONE

WHAT IS ANTIVIRALS

Antivirals are regarded or described as any compound that fights or combats viruses inside the frame. Viruses can lead to a completely extreme disease that is fatal within the human gadget. Viruses are regarded to have a prime intention, and that's to gain momentum and in addition reproduce because the case can be, which is what takes place whilst an endemic infects a mobile. The moment that virus kills the inflamed mobile; it breeds or reproduces extra virus that that yield to contaminate or infect different cells. Even though the frame gadget can combat viruses on its personal, not all honestly especially if the immune device may be very low More so, there's a special medication known as Antivirals that boost the immune system in different to fight those viruses. In this book, you may be able to find out how natural herbs are Antivirals, how to prepare, its benefit, the way to use, and their safety precautions. We can, in addition, look at all-herbal antibiotics and it may be applied to yield a satisfactory result.

CHAPTER TWO

WHY CHOOSE A NATURAL ANTIVIRALS AND ATIBIOTICS

Antibiotics are used to kill or inhibit bacteria boom. Despite the fact which you might imagine approximately antibiotics as a present-day medication, they've in fact been around for centuries. The particular antibiotics, like a variety of in recent times' antibiotics, are derived from herbal resources.

Certain plant extracts, vital oils, or even food have antibiotic homes. For instance, some meals and vegetable extracts can save you the boom of bacteria in meals.

Every so often, those houses make bigger past the food and can use sources in your non-public hygiene. Cranberry extract incorporates every antibacterial and antioxidant compound, making it a home cure for urinary tract infections (UTIs).

Herbs can be antibiotics, too. A small sampling look at 58 Chinese language flowers decided that 23 had antibacterial properties and 15 had antifungal houses.

A 2014 look at relied on supply observed that a natural remedy modified into surely as effective as a chemical antibiotic in treating a small intestine bacterial overgrowth disorder.

The use of Honey:

Honey is one of the oldest regarded antibiotics, tracing lower back to ancient times.

Honey incorporates hydrogen peroxide relied on supply, which may additionally account for a number of its antibacterial residences. It additionally has an immoderate sugar content material, which could assist prevent the boom of sure microorganisms.

Additionally, honey has a low pH level. This works to drag moisture away from a microorganism, inflicting the microorganism to get dehydrated and die off.

To apply honey as an antibiotic, follow it right now to the wound or infected place. The honey can assist kill off the microorganism and useful aid within the recovery way. If feasible, choose raw Manuka honey. This form of honey offers maximum fitness benefits. You should buy raw Manuka honey here.

You can moreover ingest honey to aid in the treatment of inner infections. Without a doubt swallow an entire tablespoon or stir it proper right into a heat cup of natural tea for a chilled deal with.

Honey is normally cozy to use at the pores and skin or inside the frame, although you have to in no way supply honey to a toddler underneath 1-12 months antique. Rather, seek advice from your healthcare provider for the great opportunity.

Using Garlic extract:

Garlic has long been the idea to have antimicrobial houses. 2011 takes a look at positioned that garlic will pay attention to is effective in opposition to microorganisms. You can purchase garlic pay interest or extract at your neighborhood fitness meals maintain. You can additionally be able to make your very personal via soaking a few garlic cloves in olive oil.

Garlic is commonly secure to ingest, however, huge doses would possibly motive internal bleeding. Up to two cloves constant with the day is considered a suitable dosage. in case you're taking a garlic supplement, make sure to comply with the dosage instructions as supplied.

In case you're taking a blood-thinning remedy, are seeking advice from your healthcare provider earlier than using garlic as an antibiotic. big doses of garlic can amplify the results of this remedy.

You could also comply with garlic listen right now to a wound or blemish.

The usage of Myrrh extract:

Many human beings are familiar with myrrh, but, its ability to keep off harmful germs isn't as widely known.

Researchers in a 2000 study concluded that an extract of myrrh should kill off numerous normal pathogens. This consists of:

Staphylococcus aureus

Pseudomonas aeruginosa

Candida albicans

Myrrh is normally well-tolerated, however eating it could motive diarrhea. If utilizing myrrh to the pores and skin, it's possible to enjoy a small pore and skin rash. If consumed in large doses, myrrh may also reason heart troubles.

Myrrh is usually prepackaged, so make certain to observe the dosage commands at the label.

The use of Thyme essential oil:

Many all-herbal family cleaners use thyme essential oil. This oil has been shown to be especially helpful toward antibiotic-resistant microorganisms.

In a 2011 examination relied on supply, researchers tested the effectiveness of each lavender and thyme crucial oil every of the oil was examined in a pool of over one hundred twenty traces of microorganism. The researchers observed thyme critical oil to be greater powerful at killing bacteria than lavender essential oil.

Thyme critical oil is for external use most effective. You shouldn't take thyme oil through the mouth. Earlier than using the affected vicinity, be sure to dilute the crucial oil with equal factors provider oil. Commonplace issuer oils encompass coconut and olive oils.

Applying undiluted critical oil to the pores and skin might also purpose infection and irritation.

Humans with excessive blood pressure or hyperthyroid troubles shouldn't use thyme essential oil.

The usage of Oregano critical oil:

Carvacrol is a detail located in oregano critical oil. It has critical therapeutic houses that further prompt restoration inside the frame while inhaling. Oregano oil has been found to help heal gastric ulcers and decrease contamination.

To cope with fungal infections to your pores and skin, add one drop of oregano important oil consistent with a teaspoon of service oil including olive or coconut oil. Take a look at the aggregate to the affected region.

You could moreover diffuse oregano oil in the air to help clear sinus infections. You shouldn't ingest oregano vital oil or use undiluted crucial oil at the pores and pores and skin.

You may moreover be able to eliminate microorganism within the domestic with a homemade cleaning agent made from:

Oregano important oil

Vinegar

Water

Lemon

The use of Echinacea:

Echinacea is a type of daisy flower it really is regularly determined inside the Japanese and crucial components of North the USA. Those flower extracts and pastes are been used for the remedy of diverse infections for the cause that early cultures. Echinacea extracts at the moment are wide to be had throughout the globe and its antimicrobial features are being utilized by humans around the world in a completely positive way. The

Immuno-shielding detail of this drug additionally makes it rather beneficial and endorsed to be protected inside the treatment of severe scientific conditions.

Echinacea has many benefits that come because of its easy components of carbohydrates, glycoprotein, and caffeic acid. These compounds have high-quality antibacterial and fungal homes and are mainly useful in reducing the spread and increase of those harmful microbes. This herb is likewise effective in reducing the issues triggered due to the signs of bacterial infections through the usage of reducing the producing cytokines that act as inflammatory markers all through an event of infection.

The usage of pink Pepper:

Crimson pepper is usually called as capsicum in other elements of the area. There are various versions of red pepper which include cayenne, chili, and jalapenos. The prevalence of pepper is found in many one-of-a-kind parts of the area aside from South the USA. They'll be blessed with masses of antibacterial homes that could assist in making the microbes disappear from the website on-line of contamination.

Capsaicin is the compound that offers pepper the spice; it additionally enables in decreasing the pH of the stomach and thereby prevents harmful bacteria from growing. Other compounds found in peppers collectively with quercetin, kaempferol, and caffeic acid has an innate capacity to stiffen the outer layer of the bacteria and thereby region a block to any and all absorption of power thereby killing it.

The use of Tea Tree Oil:

Don't be careworn tea tree oil isn't always made from the tea flowers from which fit to be eaten tea leaves are cultivated, as a substitute, tea tree is an indigenous tree it's positioned within the continent of Australia and New Zealand. The extract taken from this tea is pretty poisonous and may reason severe issues if fed on orally. Tea tree oil also is going by means of manner of the call of melaleuca oil in some additives of the arena.

Tea tree oil is wealthy in compounds in conjunction with monoterpenes which are very effective in preventing the direction of microorganisms. This compound has the potential to inhibit the sports activities of herpes virus and make your stay comfortable with those sorts of deadly infections. You ought to continuously recollect to no longer practice tea tree oil in the centered shape as this can motive many pores and skin problems. Tea tree oil is simplest allowed to be carried out in its diluted layout because of its immoderate consciousness of herbal bureaucracy.

The use of Turmeric:

Turmeric is an Indian spice that is regarded for its antimicrobial homes. The usage of turmeric may be very sturdy and obtrusive in the Indian way of existence. Referred to as Haldi, there can be an actual purification occasion for the bride which incorporates the usage of haldi to keep her pure from pores and skin-based totally infections. Turmeric is also appreciably utilized in lots of Indian dishes for its flavor and antimicrobial results.

Curcumin is the liveliest detail in turmeric and it gives an entire lot of blessings on your body. Curcumin is very effective in treating UTI (Urinary Tract Infections) because it has some very effective abilities in lowering the hobby of the microbes causing the infection.

The anti-inflammatory homes of curcumin make turmeric very powerful in treating conditions induced because of belly inflammations. Turmeric also can characteristic nicely with antibiotics lowering the harmful effects of the latter; research has shown that once turmeric is used at the side of antibiotics it could lessen the inflammatory effects at the lungs. Turmeric is also famous for its consequences at the fantastically risky HIV virus and moreover for its capability to forestall the replication of the hepatitis C virus.

Using Clove:

Clove is virtually a well-known spice utilized in huge amounts spherical in the arena. by and large, determined in Asia, cloves have a tremendous antimicrobial home which makes it a notable spice. It's widely utilized in maximum Indian dishes, because of the particular taste it provides to the food.

Cloves are rich in Eugenol which gives it wonderful antibacterial residences that may help in making you secure from unwanted bacterial infections. Cloves additionally have the capability to damage the overlying layers of bacterial cells as a result of blocking off the manufacturing of protein and

DNA which could prove deadly for the survival of the microorganism.

Oral candidacies also can be avoided by way of eating cloves orally as this may actively save you the website hosting and spread of Candida Albicans species of fungi, the taste that cloves add for your meals makes it easy to be consumed. The flexibility of cloves can test in diverse dishes in which you can additionally enjoy the antimicrobial houses of this spice.

The use of Thyme:

Thyme is a well-known spice at the completely used inside the Mediterranean cuisine. The antimicrobial traits of this spice are very immoderate. it may be without trouble be inculcated in numerous dishes and might provide multiple advantages to your frame.

Thyme can be extracted from its oil and this oil can be very effective to deal with illnesses brought about because of Escheria Coli and Pseudomonas aeruginosa bacterias.

It can actively prevent the functioning of these quorum sensing organisms without posing an awful lot of harm to your body because of facet consequences. Thyme extracts also are very powerful in treating conditions that are induced because of the effects of herpes viruses.

The usage of Lemongrass:

Lemongrass is a well-known detail around the area. The particular aroma of lemongrass makes it quite used in dishwashing soaps and different hygienic merchandise. Yet every different reason at the back of that is the fact lemongrass has terrific antibacterial, antifungal, and antiviral houses.

Citral alpha and citral beta compounds determined in lemongrass are responsible for the functionality it has in blocking extensive spectrum bacteria within the format of lemongrass oil. Lemongrass oil is rather useful in handling staph and salmonella microorganisms and additionally e-coli without causing numerous aspect outcomes, in contrast to antibiotics that have many aspect results.

In a test performed on guinea pigs, lemongrass extract application modified into useful in reducing the effects of ringworm infection at the pores and pores and skin. Lemongrass oil is likewise effective against candidacies as it is able to inhibit the number one feature of the fungus. An additional terrific benefit of this herbal antibiotic is that it can prevent the replication of the HIV virus by way of reducing the function of HIV-1 TAT protein.

Using Rosemary:

Rosemary is a totally common herb that is used inside the education of many food merchandises around the sector. Rosemary has incredible antiviral, antibacterial, and anti-fungal houses which makes it considerably useful for human consumption.

Rosemary is rich in compounds like alpha-pinene, camphene, alpha-terpinol, 1, and eight cineole and borneol. Those compounds are noticeably effective in treating conditions together with viral infections and cancer. The anti-oxidizing person of this herb will assist in making the intake enables in stopping the external forces of oxidation that may be dangerous on your frame.

Rosemary is a completely powerful natural antibiotic without facet-effects in treating conditions including salmonella infections and staph infections; it was given super outcomes in stopping quorum sensing bacterias. Rosemary is likewise famous for its antiviral capabilities in fighting the HIV-R virus. Ingesting rosemary can each make your meals and live healthy and fun.

The usage of natural antibiotics, instead of western medicine, can maximum correctly gain you ultimately. Antibiotics take a heavy toll on the organs and the herbal skills of the body and can also purpose the collateral destruction of ideal bacterias which are desired to your intestines. The unfavorable side effects of antibiotics can, consequently, be really eradicated through the substitution of natural antibiotics. But, it's also recommended that you do now not keep on natural remedy if the signs and symptoms and symptoms do no longer disappear with use, you want to be careful and seek advice from a doctor immediately.

CONCLUSION

At this period when there are lots of viral illnesses everywhere in the globe, the ones which are regarded and those that aren't yet located. In essence, we must stay guided. What I mean is that understanding the primary preparations of herbal roots which might be inside our reach is critical for our health in some unspecified time in the future while the need arises. Each medicine, name it English remedy as we fondly appear it is has a grass root foundation. Herbal medication can stand the flavor of the time and assist build our gadget hormones sooner or later in time. We ought to take it very extreme for a better healthier dwelling for now not just ourselves, but also, our cherished ones and family at massive.

There's no virus that could stand a better rooted natural medicinal drug when nicely made.

As I have said upward. Examine cautiously and now not just analyzing, exercise it for that reason.

www.ingramcontent.com/pod-product-compliance
Lightning Source LLC
Chambersburg PA
CBHW050756250726
48662CB00005B/2244